It Doesn't Have to Be Green

Your Collection of Super-Healthy, Tasty, Non-Green Alkaline Juices for Energy and Vitality

By Marta "Wellness" Tuchowska
Copyright ©Marta Tuchowska 2019

ISBN: 978-1672272506

All information in this book has been carefully researched and checked for factual accuracy. However, the author and publishers make no warranty, expressed or implied, that the information contained herein is appropriate for every individual, situation or purpose, and assume no responsibility for any errors or omissions.

The reader assumes the risk and full responsibility for all actions and the author will not be held liable for any loss or damage, whether consequential, incidental, and special or otherwise, that may result from the information presented in this publication.

The book is not intended to provide medical or professional advice or to take the place of medical/professional advice and treatment from your personal physician. Readers are advised to consult their doctors or other qualified health professionals regarding the treatment of medical conditions.

The author shall not be held liable or responsible for any misunderstanding or misuse of the information contained in this book. The information is not intended to diagnose, treat or cure any disease.

Contents

Don't Like Juicing Greens?

We've Got You Covered!

Welcome to *It Doesn't Have to Be Green, AKA (Alkaline) Juicing for People Who Hate Greens...*

The goal of this book is to teach you how to make super-healthy, healing, nutrient-packed juices without using greens.

And I want to show you how much variety you can put into non-green alkaline juicing so that you can take meaningful action and feel confident that you are getting closer to your health goals. If you want to enjoy more energy and vitality and give your body what it needs to thrive, you have come to the right place.

Through this book, you will quickly discover what most people overlook on their health journeys...heck, you will even find out what many "seasoned health freaks" overlook.

I will also be very transparent about my own mistakes so that you can avoid them and focus on what really works for you and your journey!

And yes, you can make amazingly healthy alkaline juices without using greens.

Besides, not all green foods (or drinks) are automatically alkaline. And not all alkaline foods have to be green.

Yes, I know it all may sound a bit confusing, especially if you are new to this, but don't worry. I will teach you everything you need to know about enjoying an alkaline diet and foods (natural and practical to follow). After reading this book, you will know exactly what to do to enhance your lifestyle and diet with the power of alkaline foods (in alignment with your nutritional choices, because everyone is different).

But before we dive deeper into the role of alkaline foods...first things first...

I want to make one thing clear- I am not against green foods. And I am not against juicing them. In fact, I love my leafy greens. And they love me too (at least I hope so!).

I love my green salads, juices, and smoothies and I have already devoted quite a few books to them.

When it comes to greens, I don't have any problem with them. I consider myself lucky in that regard. But not everyone is the same.

Yes, Generally Speaking, Greens Are Good for You, But...

Some people have to stay away from leafy greens because of allergies or some medical conditions.

Even the healthiest green superfoods that work great for most people may not be suitable for everyone.

I am like a broken record with that. And even though I am a big fan of green foods, the number one thing when creating your own diet should be -your unique individual situation.

And there will always be some foods that disagree with you. Perhaps you have already been to doctors, dieticians, and naturopaths and know which foods you need to avoid. And some of these foods maybe be super-healthy green foods. But they are not made for you, and that is okay.

You can let them go as there will always be other options for you.

Last year it became clear to me that I had more and more readers who, for some reason, had to let go of eating and drinking greens. Greens did not serve them well.

And they thought they could no longer live an alkaline lifestyle because of that.

Luckily, there are many other super-healthy, non-green ingredients you can juice, and this is why I am writing this book.

At first, I did a little experiment last year when I created my an online course related to alkaline lifestyle. Inside that course, I included a little bonus called *Alkaline Juicing for People Who Hate Greens.* It was supposed to be a test, and I just had this intuitive feeling it was the right thing to create for the clients of my course.

People loved it. And so, a few weeks before writing this book, I began sharing some non-green juicing recipes on my blog and via my email newsletters.

And more and more people loved it.

I also noticed that some people simply didn't like greens. They felt put off by them. They just didn't like the color and found it hard to be drinking something green (even if the recipe itself was tasty and balanced).

Some people, on the other hand, myself included, were looking for a variety of different options. I love greens. But I like other colors too. I love balance, abundance, and variety.

And this is what I am absolutely passionate about- I love giving people different options. So, even if you are a green juice monster, you can still enjoy a variety of balanced, colorful, low-sugar, and nutrient-packed (aka alkaline) juices.

Yes- talking about juices and drinks...everything that is very low in sugar, high in nutrients, caffeine-free, gluten-free, and lactose-free (all at the same time) is alkaline (to keep things simple for now). Later, in this book, I will explain more about the alkaline diet.

Why I Wrote This Book

Well, by now, I guess it's pretty obvious. I wanted to give you different options and stimulate your "outside the box" thinking so that you feel empowered knowing how much variety you can put into super-healthy, alkaline juicing.

My goal behind creating this book is to give you actionable information, motivation, and inspiration to help you take action and experience real holistic transformation.

You will then be able to enjoy more energy, vitality, and zest for life and use your health transformation to achieve all your other life goals. It all starts with health and vibrant energy.

Juicing Offers a Myriad of Benefits

The whole idea behind juicing is to provide rest for your digestive tract and the organs responsible for digestion, energy production, and waste control (kidneys, bladder, colon, liver, intestines), thereby, helping you achieve a healthier digestive system.

Aside from the actual "rest" for your digestive system, you are also feeding your body with a myriad of nutrients to help your body heal faster and feel amazing.

When you juice your foods, you take all the fiber out of it, which leaves room for the *instant absorption* of nutrients and faster conversion of food to energy in the blood.

(By the way, you can still keep the fiber and add it to your salads, plant-based stir-fries, or even healthy, gluten-free baking recipes, if you wish.)

When you drink fresh alkaline juices, you will have more stamina and energy, simply because your body will utilize the saved energy derived from digestion and conversion of food to blood sugar.

Almost 30% of the energy in the body can be used for other activities. Fresh, alkaline juice is the best natural "coffee" for your body and mind. And it truly has the power to revitalize all the systems your body needs to pay you back with vibrant health.

The fact that nutrients are quickly absorbed from juice means they are distributed rapidly to cells, thereby aiding healing and repairs.

Antioxidants derived from alkaline foods that are easily accessible have the potential to swiftly reduce damage brought about by free radicals and lessen the risk of many preventable diseases.

Whether you are new to juicing or are already seasoned and are just looking for new recipes and inspiration- you have come to the right place. I intend to give you tools and motivation so that you can use juicing as a natural therapy to help you create a healthier and stronger version of yourself.

This is what we will be covering, step-by-step:

1.JUICING MISTAKES TO AVOID

First, I want to make sure you juice the RIGHT way so that you can experience all the benefits of juicing for years to come. So, I will be the first one to share my early juicing mistakes…Luckily for you, you will be equipped with proven information and quality recipes, so you will not make those mistakes…

However, I still want to be sure you understand how it works so that you feel empowered and confident knowing that you can create your own juicing recipes that are healthy and balanced.

They say that taking any action is better than taking no action. Well, it depends. This can be true when it comes to "paralysis analysis" kind of situation. For example, people getting a ton of books and courses without taking action because it's all too confusing. (I have been guilty of that for sure!) But, when it comes to improving your wellbeing, why not focus on taking the right action? That doesn't mean you have to be perfect. All you need is to have a healthy foundation…

2.MANAGING YOUR GOALS AND EXPECTATIONS

Yes, I know, not very sexy! But I genuinely believe you need to know how to manage your expectations. When I first got started on helping people improve their wellbeing, I thought it was enough for me to give them my information, and then they would somehow stick to it and get results. But, very soon I realized that I had to learn more about mindset, psychology, and how our minds can easily get brainwashed by what is out there.

I quickly realized that some people who came to me for help had very unrealistic expectations that they got from some hype health and fitness gurus.

Juicing is not a magical overnight cure. It is merely a tool and natural therapy. It requires commitment and needs to be backed up with solid, healthy lifestyle choices.

This is precisely what I will be helping you with through this book. This is what "holistic" really means. It's not as simple as going for something natural (or expecting an overnight result from "something natural"). It's about integrating all your systems, mind, body, and soul and becoming a stronger person as a result.

3. WHAT IS "ALKALINE"? IS IT SAFE? ISN'T IT ANOTHER HEALTH HYPE?

I am a big fan of alkaline foods and drinks, and in case you are new to the alkaline lifestyle, I will give you a rapid crash course so that you know what it is and how it works.

The solid foundation I will give you will help you understand which foods are alkaline, even without needing any alkaline charts and food lists. I will also share with you a straightforward and intuitive way of alkaline eating.

Oh, and since it's a book on juicing, you will also learn why alkaline foods are the best foods to focus on when juicing and why it's got more to do with what those foods consist of and their nutritional value (and not about their pH).

We will also debunk the most common alkaline myths that are being spread by hype gurus. Understanding that part is the most crucial piece of this juicing puzzle. Well, all of them are important since we are thinking holistically here.

Trust me...reading those few pages alone will be of huge help for you and your loved ones, and when applied consistently the principles can really help you transform your wellbeing.

4. TOOLS, EQUIPMENT, AND SUPPLEMENTS NEEDED FOR THIS STYLE OF JUICING.

In this section, I will cover the best juicers for a super healthy juicing and other tools/ products you may find beneficial. Remember, though, the most important thing is your favorite juicer and your commitment to using it.

The simpler you keep it, the better. As one of my mentors once told me, to succeed at anything and maintain that success, you need a simple process. It should consist of three basic moves. All you need to focus on is repetition.

For example, let's say your goal is to have more energy. Well, a simple process to begin with, could look like this:

1. Have a nutritious smoothie for breakfast.

2. Serve your lunch with a big bowl of salad.

3. In the afternoon, instead of going for another coffee to keep going, have some fresh, alkaline juice.

These three simple actions can get you fantastic and sustainable results...but it all comes down to consistency.

Yea, I know, not very sexy! Especially because our brains are designed to rebel and resist. We love going after what is new, and we love the dopamine release that comes with "trying out something new." Well, to achieve new results and to really transform, it's essential to be patient and focus on the process.

5. FINALLY...NON-GREEN JUICING FOOD LISTS

This one will be easy after all the positive, alkaline-friendly "brainwashing" from the section on alkaline diet and foods. The list of foods will still be abundant and will make so much sense, enabling you to prepare super healthy, colorful, nutritious juices you will love!

6. And then, the recipes and THEY LIVED HAPPILY EVER AFTER!

My intention is not just to throw some recipes at you. The recipes I create are like living beings to me, and I want you to make friends with them. Before you even meet them, though, I want you to know what they're like and if you should hang out together, why and when.

To keep it simple- I have done all the thinking and homework for you, so all you need to do it to take action, incorporate those recipes into your lifestyle, and let the juicing transform you from the inside out.

Then, if you decide to write me a review or a testimonial, I will feel like it's well deserved, and that we both worked hard for it and we can help and inspire other people.

Otherwise, the transformation we go through can be lonely and boring.

By choosing to shine and be the best versions of ourselves, we also get to motivate and inspire other people. Not necessarily by speaking on the most famous stages of the world but by choosing to be courageous and unique in our everyday actions. Doing things a little bit differently and setting an example for other people to follow.

It can help many people improve not only their quality of life but also avoid many preventable diseases. How great is that?

Let's do this, we are in this together, and I am really looking forward to guiding you through each step covered in this book.

It all starts with HEALTH

You have the choice to get closer to the health, vitality, strength, fitness, spirituality, and abundance of your dreams by taking small (but firm) baby steps every day.

Think about all the areas of your life:

Your family and loved ones...

Your passions and hobbies...

Your work, career, and job/business...

Your stamina, strength, fitness...

How you feel and how you look...

All these areas depend on how you show up, your courage, energy, and vitality. By working on your energy (this book will show you how to do it on a physical level), you will automatically feel more motivated. And people love motivated people- it's infectious!

Besides, by making a choice to get healthier, you are working not only on your energy and vitality but also on your character, your discipline, and your mindset...

You can then use your health, power, and "holistic strength" to fuel all areas of your life...

Re-read this page whenever you get off track and need inspiration. Some days you will feel off or less motivated. But do not let some temporary low feelings stop you.

Acknowledge them and keep going because you are a true holistic warrior.

Juicing Mistakes to Avoid

If you are reading this book, I assume you already know the difference between juicing and making smoothies.

But just in case you are new to this...

It's not uncommon to put smoothies and juices in the same categories- "Oh, just some healthy juices." However, smoothies are not the same as juices. Smoothies are made by blending fruits and veggies (using a blender or a food processor).

In that process, all the fiber remains intact. You can also blend in some nuts and seeds or protein powder. This means that a smoothie can be made as a quick and healthy meal replacement (as long as it is satisfying, nutritious as well as rich in protein and good fats).

When it comes to juicing, though- we don't blend. We extract. As a result, there is no fiber. Only pure, super-easy, and quick to digest juice.

Both smoothies and juices are fantastic. It's not that juices are better than smoothies, or smoothies better than juices.

Everything depends on everything else, and both juices and smoothies must be done the right way.

So, when it comes to juices, here are some common mistakes:

1. Some people think they can have a juice as a meal replacement, or they exaggerate with very strict juice cleanses to lose weight fast.

In reality, to be more effective, juicing is a natural therapy that should be combined with a clean and nutritionally balanced unprocessed food diet. It's not about going hungry and starving yourself on some juices. Yes, you could lose some weight fast only to confuse your body later and put it all back on again.

My stand on juicing is this: use it as an additional, natural, and holistic therapy to help you have more energy and combine it with a healthy, balanced, clean food diet that suits you and your personal needs.

So, if your goal is to lose weight healthily and sustainably (whether you are a young female or not), please do yourself a favor and focus on abundance. An abundance of nutrients. Don't deprive yourself of food. Just eat clean. Add fresh juices, as recommended in this book, as a tool to help your body thrive by adding in a ton of easy to digest nutrients. Be patient and keep going. Not only will you transform your body but also your mindset and your emotions.

At the same time, I am not bashing juice cleanses. But my work is not aimed at using juicing for prolonged juice cleanses. If you would like to do a juice cleanse, I would highly recommend you consult with a naturopathic doctor to make sure such a cleanse is the right thing for you to do.

The most balanced, most comfortable to stick to, and most common-sense thing to do, is to clean up your diet and add fresh juices on top of that. No starvation. Eat more. But eat real, nutrient-packed foods. Your body loves real food. Oh, and some juicing.

Ok, so that was mistake number one- using juices as a meal replacement or going through unrealistic, starvation cleanses to lose weight fast.

2. The second mistake is not knowing what to juice for optimal benefits.

We have already covered the difference between smoothies and juices. When drinking a smoothie, you also get the fiber from the fruits and veggies you blended.

However, juices are extracts and elixirs, and there is no fiber in them. This is why it's super important to avoid juicing fruit that is high in sugar.

Yes, avoid high sugar fruit juice, even fresh. Fruit that is higher in sugar is much better eaten as a whole or blended in a smoothie.

To make sure you juice the right way, you want to focus on low sugar ingredients- and this is what this book will show you how to do.

That little shift alone can help you massively boost your wellbeing. Also, it's good to know you don't need to buy a ton of super expensive, exotic fruit to do your juicing. By focusing on low-sugar ingredients, not only will it be easier to find all the ingredients you need, it will be less expensive, and what's most important- very healthy.

So, yes- fresh, whole fruit, for example, apple, pears, pineapple, kiwis, etc. are good as a quick snack, or maybe a little addition to your smoothies to make them taste nice. But remember that drinking fruit juices is like drinking pure sugar.

Processed fruit juices with all the added sugar and chemicals on top of that are even worse.

(Of course, an occasional exception, like adding a bit of apple to your green spinach juice, or maybe some orange to your kale juice is not a crime- but for the sake of this book, since we are focusing on non-green, you will learn how to make super-healthy juices using low sugar fruit and other excellent superfood ingredients).

If you are a curious soul (like I am) and what I have written above is not enough to convince you, here's what happens when we drink fruit juice made of high sugar fruit:

When you remove the fiber, the liquid juice is absorbed into your bloodstream much quicker than it does with fiber.

This is why, if you are juicing fruits, it will lead to unstable blood sugar levels and a drop in blood sugar. This can cause low energy levels and sugar cravings. Drinking pure fruit juices will make you hungry, and your body will ask for more sugar to add to the vicious cycle.

And so, because of that, the "juicing haters" are right. When it comes to high sugar fruit, keep that fiber intact and make a smoothie instead of a juice. Your body will tell you when to stop because there is a limit to how much fiber-rich smoothie you can drink.

If you want to juice the right way- go for low sugar ingredients. It's as simple as that.

Also, not everyone can handle smoothies. Some people can't tolerate too much fiber (even natural fiber). Juicing is recommended for those who have a sensitive digestive system or illness that inhibits your body from processing fiber. Since there is no fiber, you only get nutrients, and your body does not need extra energy to digest it.

Managing Your Juicing Goals and Expectations

Now, it's time to manage your expectations. I am sure you are excited about juicing, and you should be. When done consistently (yes, the keyword here is *consistency*) and the right way, it can really boost your wellbeing and help you stay healthy.

It all depends on where you are on your journey right now. If you are already eating clean, scheduling self-care, moving your body, and working on your mindset, etc. then adding some healthy juicing will help you optimize what you are already doing. All the hard work you put in will get amplified. You will manifest amazing results.

And so, you may start feeling amazing in just a few days. Your body is already in a clean, healthy state, and you are using juicing to take it to the next level.

But, if you are just starting out, be kind on yourself. Be patient and don't give up, just because you have tried a few juices and didn't feel that much of a difference.

Rome wasn't built in a day. Don't compare yourself with other people who have been on this journey longer. Instead, use them as an inspiration to help you strengthen your vision and your motivation.

Instead, look at yourself holistically. What else can you improve to make sure your juicing efforts can help your health and wellness goals?

When I say holistically, I am not only referring to "natural." Yes, holistic and natural very often overlap but I don't like using words *holistic* and *natural* interchangeably as if they were the same word because they are not.

When I say *holistically,* I mean- integrating all the systems. Your mind and soul included.

You can allow yourself to see the bigger picture of your health journey. Think where you will be in five years or ten years from now. Most importantly, think how your new, healthy mindset will help you achieve success in all areas of life.

It all starts with health, but it doesn't end there. So, use your energy and health to get closer to your life, family, and career goals too.

Some days you will feel like it doesn't make any sense. You will have those voices in your head telling you to juice tomorrow. And, you will still get up, with courage. You will still make a decision to set up your juicer and feed your body with a ton of nutrients.

I am telling it like it is. We will be climbing the health Kilimanjaro here, and some days will be tough. I want you to keep going so that you embrace and enjoy the process. Fuse yourself with your goals. Transform your self-image. If you're going to be vibrant, healthy, slim, and energized then listen to your higher self and take those healthy actions here and now, even though you are still not experiencing all the results you want to experience. They will come.

There are no quick fixes. I am like a broken record with that.

The best thing we can do is to commit to the process of taking small, consistent actions for years to come.

Don't get me wrong, you certainly don't need to wait for years to experience the energizing benefits of healthy juicing. Although, if you commit to living a healthy lifestyle, in 5 years you will be a totally new person, you will look back at your photos from now and will be grateful for the actions you have taken.

So, back to managing your expectations. You need to understand that your body, mind, and soul work as a whole. That is a holistic approach, and profound transformations do take time.

By committing to a process, you create a stronger version of yourself. Not only health-wise but also character-wise. So, by investing your time in regular juicing, you can master your motivation, discipline, and create a new self-image of someone who takes meaningful action.

You can then apply the same process to other areas of your life because taking action will be a part of who you are.

Some days, you will not feel like setting up your juicer. You will not feel like juicing. I can honestly tell you that some days, I am not motivated, and I don't feel like it.

It's like two different Martas talking to each other. Angel and devil!

You will need to become a Thought Hunter and spot those patterns right away and then say to yourself, OK, Mr. Devil, I am doing my juicing, thank you for your opinion, but I will do it anyway!

Some days, you will fall off track- and I can tell you it has happened to me too. When it does happen, it's easy to allow in self-guilt and self-pity...

"Oh, but other people on social media are so healthy, and they always post this and that..."

Yes, the online world is a different thing. It doesn't reflect the real battle that, let's face it, all of us humans can face.

And since, authenticity and honesty are a big part of my values, and I base my brand around my values, I am the first one to share what it really takes...the good and the bad.

Not to discourage you, but to help you be prepared.

So that you are not a Worry-ier but a Warrior. A real, holistic warrior who can always get back on track!

So, even before you get into the recipes from this book, ask yourself- what is a realistic commitment for you?

If you can juice every day, wow, you will feel the results. But, if you are very busy, you can also juice every other day, or set up your "juicing time" 3 times a week.

Let's be honest here. Juicing is more time consuming than making smoothies. It is what it is. But you can be proactive. You can organize your routine in a way that best suits your lifestyle.

Usually, I schedule in 3-4 juicing afternoons or evenings a week. And when I make my juice and set everything up, I like to batch juice, so that way, I also have a serving of incredibly nutritious juice for the following day.

You can also go hardcore in and juice more and juice every day. Of course, juicing should be combined with a balanced, healthy lifestyle and healthy, clean food. Yes, I know, I am repeating myself.

You see, I have come across individuals who were sporadically juicing hardcore and doing some weird juice cleanses, while still eating processed fast food. That is not balanced, and, in this case, juicing will not be effective.

However, I am positive you can start cleaning up your diet. (Juicing will also help you with that because a nourished body has fewer bad cravings.). Take it step by step and set up a regular juicing routine that is easy to stick to. Your body loves juicing and all the benefits it provides. It will start feeling clean and balanced and you will start craving real, fresh foods as a result.

So, keep moving forward and be patient.

However, if you are planning a strict juice cleanse (not something I cover in my books), I would highly recommend that you talk about it with your healthcare provider or a qualified naturopathic doctor to make sure you do the cleanse that best suits your health and your needs.

At the same time, if every now and then you skip a meal and use a juice instead, because you feel you need to give your digestive system a big rest, go for it. Sometimes I like to have an early night and substitute my regular dinner with a big, nutritious juice.

Usually, I do it when I really need to restore my energy levels and get more rest. Then, I wake up feeling refreshed and have a beautiful, healthy breakfast.

However, any strict juice cleanses should be discussed with a specialist, especially if you are suffering from any medical conditions.

Alkaline? What Is It?

I am sure you have been waiting for this! Since the book has the word "Alkaline" in the subtitle, and I have been throwing this word around quite a lot in this book, I am sure you have been expecting me to write a little bit about the pH. It's a really hot topic these days, and as with anything hot, there will always be some hype around it. And hype can create confusion. You may be thinking that you need a ton of supplements or who knows what to get closer to living a healthy, alkaline lifestyle.

The good news is that it's not as complicated as many gurus want us to believe. In fact, it's pretty common sense, healthy eating knowledge aimed at cleaning up your diet and making most of your diet rich in unprocessed and nutrient-packed foods with no nasty chemicals in them.

At the same time, eating more alkaline is a great, natural tool that can boost your immune system. It also has the potential to help you avoid many preventable diseases or recover from them faster.

Again, "going alkaline" is not a quick fix. Being unhealthy and neglecting your body for years takes some recovery. I am not judging; on my wellness journey I had to learn to be patient. So, I understand how it feels.

True transformation is based on courage, consistency, mindset, self-love, and of course, some useful information. In this case, some recommendations based on the alkaline diet and lifestyle.

Here is how it works...

The pH of most of our crucial cellular and other body fluids, like blood, is designed to be at a pH of 7.365, which is slightly alkaline.

Luckily, our miraculous body has an intricate system in place to maintain that healthy, slightly alkaline pH level. It's working for us 24/7, to ensure our pH system stays optimally balanced.

An interesting thing is that our body, as long as it is blessed with the gift of life, will continuously keep working to regulate our pH (whether we eat a healthy diet rich in alkaline foods or not).

The problem? It's up to us to make it easier or harder for our bodies...

We can totally choose what we eat. But...

If we focus on unhealthy choices, for example, the Standard Western Diet (with its overload of sugars, processed carbohydrates, dairy, soda, too many animal products, and fast food) we make it more and more difficult for our body to stay in balance.

Some people say, "Oh, but what is the point of eating a healthy diet rich in unprocessed alkaline foods if our body regulates our pH for us?"

Yes, our body regulates our pH for us.

Alkaline skeptics like using this argument, and they are actually right. Even though I am a big fan of alkaline diet and foods, I also recognize the fact there is lots of hype and unrealistic expectations in the alkaline diet area.

Once again, the hype is designed to make people buy some quick fixes and other miraculous cures. So, once again, it comes down to managing your expectations first (as we discussed earlier).

We can't make our pH higher and higher. You see, this is not the goal of the alkaline diet. We just can't make our blood's pH more alkaline or "higher." Our body tries to work hard for us to help maintain our ideal blood pH (7.365) We can't have a pH of 8 or 9.

Well, we could, but if we did, we would be dead.
It's not about magically raising or re-modifying our body's pH level.

The focus of the alkaline diet is to give your body the nourishment and the healing tools that it needs to MAINTAIN that optimal blood pH (7.365) almost effortlessly WITHOUT making you sick, tired, and moody.

Alkaline lifestyle is a tool to help you control your physical, mental, and emotional wellbeing by CHOOSING to get closer to balance.

This is achieved by taking in healthy, balanced nutrient-rich alkaline foods (you already know these are good for you!) such as:
- unprocessed foods
- naturally gluten-free foods
- yeast-free foods
- dairy-free foods
- sugar-free foods
- wheat-free foods
- foods rich in minerals, vitamins, and chlorophyll
-plant-based foods, greens, and veggies (This book in particular skips greens, as this is a non-green party, the greens already got invited to my *Alkaline Green Smoothies* book party.)

If we do not support our bodies with healthy, balanced nutrition, we torture them with incredible stress and overload!

Yes, when the body has to continually work overtime to detoxify all of the cells and maintain our pH, it finally succumbs to disease. It still keeps working and balancing...but...it gets weaker and weaker, and we no longer get to enjoy the vibrant health and vitality of our dreams. This is when we become much more prone to disease, and there's a downward spiral of physical and mental ailments.

Let me give you a few examples of what can happen if we continuously eat an acid-forming diet (also called SAD - Standard American Diet, or Standard Western Diet) that does not support our body at all. Our body ends up sick and tired of working overtime and may manifest one or more of the following conditions:

- Chronic inflammation
- Immune and hormonal imbalance
- Lack of energy, mental fog- you go for another cup of coffee yet still feel the same. Sound familiar?
- Yeast and candida overgrowth
- Digestive damage
- Weakened bones. Our body is forced to pull minerals <u>like magnesium and calcium from our bones to maintain the alkaline balance it needs for constant healing processes.</u>

In summary, eating more alkaline foods, for example, veggies, herbs, and nutrient-packed superfoods helps support our body so that it can work for us at optimal levels.

Eating more acid-forming foods (aka processed food, fast food, sugar, soda, too many animal products, etc.) doesn't help at all.

The alkaline diet is not about magically raising or changing our pH, but about helping our body rebalance itself by supporting its natural healing functions with healthy food and drink such as alkaline-friendly juices and drinks.

The commonsense explanation is to imagine you eat a hardcore Western Diet for a month. You eat processed carbs, fast food, drink soda, and bombard your body with unhealthy fats, sugars, and way too many animal products. You don't drink enough water, and you don't move your body. Needless to say, your wellbeing will not improve, and you will begin to feel tired and will very likely have pain and inflammation. (Fair enough, if you are very young, it may take some time to develop those unhealthy symptoms, but why do that to yourself?)

Then, imagine that you focus on a clean food diet (whether it's entirely plant-based, or almost plant-based, or "mixed," but still very clean and full of alkaline foods). You eat lots of vegetables, whole foods, healthy fats, and unprocessed foods. In other words, you eat a diet rich in alkaline foods. You also drink lots of clean water and nutrient-packed smoothies with healthy alkaline vegetables and fruit.

Yes, every now and then you have a treat meal or indulge in acidity very occasionally. You know, family occasions and things of that nature. However, your overall healthy balance is so strong that your body copes well with those occasional treats. And since you feel so good on a clean diet, you don't even crave those treats you used to live for anymore.

Needless to say, by eating healthier, by eating a clean food diet and optimizing your nutrition and lifestyle, you feel better and allow your body to heal faster. You treat your body as a temple!

For example, our body also regulates our temperature for us. But...what will happen if you immerse yourself in a bath full of ice cubes for too long? How long will your body keep going and regulate your temperature for you? Everything has a limit.

We can only rely on our "health credit cards" for so long...The first step for most people is to pay off that "health debt." The second step is to make sure your alkaline bank account still has funds in it. The third step is to embrace the Health Investor mindset. Every food choice we make can be an investment, or an asset, for our long-term wellness, or it can be a distraction or a loss in "alkaline profits".

The question I ask myself every day is: *Am I getting closer to or farther away from my vision?*

The Alkaline Diet is sisters with the Clean Food Diet, Anti-Inflammatory Diet, Vegetarian Diet, Vegan Diet, Macrobiotic Diet, and the Raw Food Diet. In fact, it offers an incredible blend and the best of them all. All those diets that are more in the plant-based category.

However, what may come as a big surprise to many is that there are also many similarities with Keto and Paleo Diets. Similarly to a Paleo Diet (Paleolithic Diet), the Alkaline Diet encourages you to stay away from dairy and wheat as well as processed carbs (such as pasta, cookies, etc.).

Just like the Keto Diet, the Alkaline Diet loves good fats (predominantly in their plant-based version, although many alkaline experts also recommend quality fish oils). Also, when it comes to fruit, both alkaline and keto diets encourage you to focus mostly on low-sugar fruit (as we have already covered in *juicing mistakes*).

That is why the Alkaline Diet is not just a diet. It's a lifestyle. A nutritionally conscious, healthily flexible lifestyle that can be combined with other foods you already like and benefit from to make them work even better for you.

(Yes, there is Alkaline Plant-Based, Alkaline Almost Plant-Based, Alkaline Vegetarian, Alkaline Paleo, Alkaline Keto, Alkaline Mediterranean etc.)

This is precisely what I try to share through my message. Nope, I am not an "alkaline Nazi," or a militant "alkalarian." I like helping people create balance (while respecting their nutritional choices).

Everyone is different, so your version of an alkaline diet may be different than mine. But the healthy foundation remains the same, make the majority of your diet (ideally 70-80%) rich in alkaline-forming foods. The rest can be other foods, just be sure you still go for clean and unprocessed.

Not so hard, right?

Now, I will get back to the topic of juicing.

Tools & Equipment for Juicing (Keep It Super-Simple)

I very often get asked about the tools and equipment I use to make juices (as well as smoothies).

Well, several years ago, I invested in Omega juicer, and we still keep going. I love it, and I think it's a great brand and company. Please note, they did not pay me to plug them into this book or anything. I am a happy Omega juicer customer. Before buying an Omega juicer I tried a ton of cheap juicers and brands, and they would never last longer than a few weeks or a few months at maximum.

My personal recommendation would therefore be Omega, because it's something I am using myself and am happy about.

However, you may also go for other juicers based on the following recommendation:

-Make sure to go for cold-pressed, low-speed, masticating kind of juicers.

Non-Green Alkaline Juicing Ingredient Lists

Now it's time to have a look at what to juice to make super healthy, non-green alkaline juices...

Alkaline Fruits, Veggies & Herbs:

- Bell peppers (red and yellow)

- Lemon

- Grapefruit

- Radish

- Garlic

- Pomegranate

- Mint (for aroma)

- Basil (for aroma)

- Lime

- Horse Radish

If you are new to the alkaline diet, you are probably wondering why lemons, limes, and grapefruits are considered alkaline. Aren't they acidic based on the fact they contain citric acid?

So, the answer to this question is, yes, they are acidic as far as their taste goes. If for any reason you can't stand the taste or it disagrees with you, or you are on some medication that interferes with those ingredients, or any other reason- needless to say, skip them in your recipes.

However, even though acidic in taste, lemons and grapefruits are actually considered to be alkaline-forming once metabolized. It's all about the effect the food has after it has been metabolized.

Lemons and grapefruits are rich in vitamins and alkaline minerals yet low in sugar at the same time. This is why they are considered alkaline-forming (even though they taste acidic).

Oranges, however, are not considered alkaline, because they are more abundant in sugar than lemons, limes or grapefruits.

So, the rule of the thumb is – the alkaline diet likes low sugar ingredients. These are the healthiest for juicing anyway, based on the fact we are getting rid of fiber and high sugar fruit without fiber, is pure sugar.

Also, please note, I am not paranoid about fruit. I include all kinds of fruit in my diet (fresh, seasonal). However, fruit that is richer in sugar goes into "a non-alkaline" part of my diet, while the majority of my food (about 70-80%) remains alkaline.

For you, it may be slightly different because everyone is different. But I am pretty sure you will notice a positive shift after focusing more on low sugar fruits.

More Alkaline Juice Ingredients:

- Fennel

- Beets

- Carrots

- Ginger

- Turmeric

- Cucumber

- Zucchini

- Tomato

Turmeric and ginger can really spice up your juices.

Cucumber, even though green on the outside, is really not so green once peeled and juiced. It's excellent for optimal hydration. Happily, it's somehow managed to sneak into a non-green recipe book!

The same applies to zucchini. They're not so green when peeled.

You may be wondering about tomato - whether it's a fruit and why it's alkaline. So, yes, it is a fruit, and it's considered alkaline-forming because it's low in sugar and high in nutrients. Limes, lemons, and grapefruits share the same story. I am sure you can see some simple patterns now. Especially the low-sugar and high-nutrient profile.

I love tomatoes in smoothies and juices, and I am also a big fan of spicy juices using tomatoes.

More Ingredients for Healthy Non-Green Juicing:

- Coconut milk

- Coconut water

- Plant-based milk (almond, rice, hemp, etc.)

- Herbal infusions (mint, fennel, chamomile, etc.)

- Filtered, alkaline water

- Kukicha tea

- Rooibos tea

- Green tea, (not alkaline, can be used in small amounts though)

- White tea and red tea (they still contain caffeine)

These are a great addition to your non-green juices to make them taste great or to optimize their benefits.

For example, one of my favorite morning drinks is fresh grapefruit and ginger juice mixed with some green tea.

It's very nutritious, energizing, rich in antioxidants, and sugar-free.

Alkaline oils (optional, feel free to skip if you're on a no-oil diet for whatever reason):

- avocado oil

- flax oil

- udo's oil

- coconut oil

- olive oil (cold-pressed)

Recipes & How to Use Them (precautions included)

As with all the recipes I create, the recipes included in this book are not aimed at diagnosing or curing any severe health problems. My main goal is to inspire people to live a healthier lifestyle, and to enjoy more energy for life. The work the recipes do is mostly preventative, if possible. The whole purpose behind my brand, Holistic Wellness Project, is to help ambitious people restore their energy, balance, and zest for life. Physically, mentally, and spiritually.

Alkaline foods and eating clean for energy is one of the pillars of the integrated methodology I share and teach (others revolve around mindset and mindfulness). But they are definitely not an overnight cure. Creating a healthy lifestyle requires patience, consistency, and dedication. If you ever feel like you're getting off track, re-read the introduction to this book and remind yourself why you started.

The recipes are not set in stone and can be personalized. If you are allergic to any of the ingredients- don't use them, you will still have plenty of options to pick and choose from.

If you currently suffer from any severe health conditions, are on medication, pregnant or lactating, or recovering from any medical treatment, I would recommend you talk to your health care provider before using the recipes contained in this book.

Now, it's time to get into the recipes!

Measurements Used in the Recipes

The cup measurement I use is the American Cup measurement.

I also use it for dry ingredients. If you are new to it, let me help you.

If you don't have American Cup measures, just use a metric or imperial liquid measuring jug and fill your jug with your ingredient to the corresponding level. Here's how to go about it:

1 American Cup= 250ml= 8 fl.oz.
For example:
If a recipe calls for 1 cup of almonds, simply place your almonds into your measuring jug until it reaches the 250 ml/8oz mark.

Quite easy, right?

I know that different countries use different measurements and I wanted to make things simple for you. I have also noticed that very often those who are used to American Cup measurements complain about metric measurements and vice versa. However, if you apply what I have just explained, you will find it easy to use both.

Alkaline Juicing for People Who Hate Greens – The Recipes

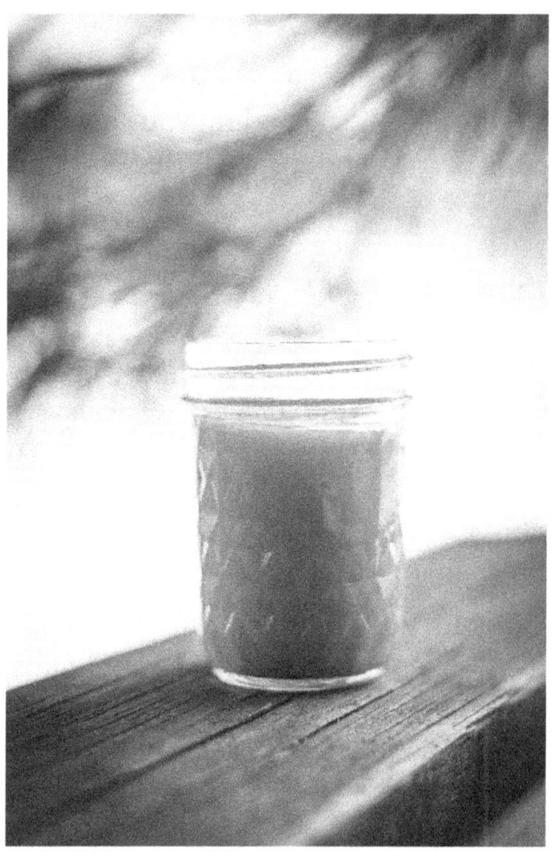

Recipe #1 "Massive Energy Injection" Juice

Avocado oil is an excellent addition to this recipe. It offers good fats to help you absorb the minerals and vitamins from the juice. I love this juice whenever I need quick and natural energy.

Himalaya salt tastes excellent in most juices, especially veggie juices or juices made with low-sugar fruit such as limes and lemons. It also adds alkaline minerals. If you like spicy juices, feel free to add in some hot sauce or chili powder.

Cucumbers are technically green, but not so green when peeled. And they don't taste green at all. They have a mild flavor, are very hydrating and super-rich in alkaline minerals. In fact, cucumbers are one of the best alkaline superfoods ever!

Servings: 1-2
Ingredients:
- 1 lemon, peeled
- 1 lime, peeled
- 2 yellow bell peppers, peeled
- 2 big cucumbers, peeled and chopped
- 1 tablespoon of avocado oil
- Himalayan salt to taste
- Optional: A couple dashes of hot habanero sauce or chili powder

Instructions:
1. Place the lemon, lime, peppers, and cucumbers in a juicer, to extract the juice.

2. Combine the juice with the avocado oil and Himalayan salt.
3. If needed, add some chili powder and/or hot sauce.
4. Serve in a glass and enjoy!

Recipe #2 "Restore Your Balance" Creamy Juice

Can juice be creamy? Well, it can undoubtedly taste creamy. This non-green juice recipe is beginner-friendly, and it's also designed to help you fight sugar cravings because of the good fats from coconut oil that it contains.

Ginger adds some anti-inflammatory properties, and it also helps strengthen your immune and digestive systems.

Serves: 1-2
Ingredients:
- 1 cup red bell peppers, seeded and chopped
- 2 carrots, peeled
- 1 lime, peeled
- 2-inch ginger, peeled
- 1 tablespoon melted coconut oil
- half cup coconut milk (unsweetened)
- optional: a pinch of cinnamon and nutmeg powder

Instructions:
1. Place the peppers, carrots, lime, and ginger in a juicer and extract the juice.
2. Pour it into a big glass.
3. Combine with coconut milk and oil.
4. Stir in the cinnamon and nutmeg powder.
5. Stir well and enjoy.

Recipe #3 "So Healthy Glow" Non-Green Juice

This recipe uses turmeric that is very alkalizing and also offers anti-inflammatory benefits.

When peeling, cutting and juicing turmeric, I recommend you use gloves (unless you want to walk around with orange nails and hands for the next 2 days, lol).

The recipe also uses carrots and other carotene-rich ingredients to help you have a beautiful, glowing, and healthy-looking skin.

Another winner for those who are not fans of juicing greens!

Servings: 2
Ingredients:
- 2 big red or yellow bell peppers, seeded and chopped
- 4 big carrots, peeled
- 2 big tomatoes, peeled
- 2 inches of turmeric, peeled (use gloves)
- Half a lemon, peeled
- 1 tablespoon avocado oil
- Pinch of black pepper
- Optional: a pinch of Himalayan salt

Instructions:
1. Juice the peppers, carrots, tomatoes, turmeric, and lemon.
2. Add in the avocado oil, pepper, and salt.
3. Serve in a glass.
4. Enjoy!

Recipe #4 "Fat-Burning Holistic Tea" Juice

The alkaline diet lifestyle is pretty much caffeine-free by design. If you balance yourself with alkaline foods and drinks, you naturally get more energy, so you don't need to rely on caffeine. Too much caffeine can lead to adrenal fatigue, mess up your digestion, and lead to tension headaches.

However, I believe that there is nothing wrong with an occasional cup of coffee or tea (black or green) as a treat.

The problem is when you need caffeine to keep you going or when you can't crawl out of bed without it. As an ex-coffee addict, I have been there. The bottom line is- *balance is the key.* I know it's not easy to get off caffeine, as you may start experiencing headaches and irritability.

This is why I offer a simple, little-by-little approach. Green tea can help you make the transition. Of course, we need to remember that green tea, even though it's green, is not fully alkaline because it still contains caffeine.

Luckily for us, green tea has some really great antioxidant and fat-burning properties and is nothing to fear. Just use it in moderation (like all kinds of caffeine-containing teas). This recipe is excellent if you get up early or need an extra energy boost.

I am actually having a cup of green tea now (I usually mix it with fennel tea to create balance, fennel tea is alkaline and caffeine-free).

You can make this recipe on the go, and you don't even need a proper juicer. In fact, you can use a simple lemon squeezer.

Servings: 1-2
Ingredients:
- half cup of green tea, cooled down (you can also mix green tea with some fennel tea), use 1 teabag per half cup water
- 2 grapefruits, juiced (you can use a lemon squeezer)
- 1 lemon, juiced (you can use a lemon squeezer)
- Optional: stevia to sweeten if needed

Instructions:
1. Make the green tea and cool it down a bit so that it's still warm, but not super-hot.
2. Mix your green tea/fennel tea with grapefruit/lemon juice.
3. Add in some stevia to sweeten, if needed.
4. Serve as it is (slightly warm) or chilled with ice cubes.
5. Enjoy your little green tea "high"!

Additional Information:
Green tea benefits:
-Better focus, concentration, and mental alertness. These benefits are not so much due to the caffeine present in green tea, but more because it is rich in a substance called L-theanine.

Green tea contains less caffeine than coffee, which is a good thing, as too much caffeine results in an energy crash.

According to the *Journal of Nutrition*, L-theanine is an amino acid that can increase the activity of the inhibitory neurotransmitter, GABA, which has anti-anxiety effects. Aside from that, it also helps release more dopamine (natural high!) and produces alpha waves in the brain (better concentration).

L-theanine works in synergy with caffeine and has been proven effective in bettering brain function.

-Fat burn and improved metabolic rate

-Less infection and better dental health. The catechins in green tea can prevent the growth of bacteria and some viruses responsible for caries, bad breath, and mouth diseases.

To sum up, if you need some caffeine in your life, green tea is a great drink. Of course, moderation is the key!

Fennel tea benefits:
-It acts as an antispasmodic, anti-inflammatory, and antibacterial/antimicrobial as its seeds are rich in crucial volatile oil compounds, like anethole, fenchone, and estragole.

-It promotes a healthier immune system, better digestion, soothes nerves, and helps you relax, and it is fantastic for digestion (it also helps alleviate PMS and bloating).

To sum up, if I were to choose only 1 herb to take with me to a desert island, it would be fennel. No doubt about it.

Recipe #5 Optimal Balance "It Doesn't Have to be Green" Juice

Beginners often complain that juicing is difficult because it calls for many exotic ingredients or ones that are difficult to find. Some complain that the alkaline lifestyle is not realistic because of that.

These complaints arise because of two things- lack of correct information as well as unrealistic expectations ingrained by media hype.

It's NOT your fault.

The truth is that juicing doesn't require any fancy fruit or exotic ingredients. You can create uncomplicated and very therapeutic juices with simple ingredients you can easily find at your local grocery store.

And these are very good for you, especially for juicing, because they are low in sugar. This juice can also be served as a quick aperitif before the main meal.

Cucumber makes a comeback in this recipe, and before anyone complains, "Oh, but it's a green veggie!"

It's not so green when naked!

Servings: 2
Ingredients:
- 4 big cucumbers, peeled and cut into smaller pieces
- 4 big tomatoes
- 1-inch ginger, peeled
- 2 big carrots, peeled and cut into smaller pieces
- 1 lemon, peeled
- Half cup water, filtered, preferably alkaline
- Pinch of Himalayan salt
- Pinch of black pepper

Instructions:
1. Juice the cucumbers, tomatoes, ginger, carrots, and lemon.
2. Combine the fresh juice with some water.
3. Stir well, drink, and enjoy!

Tomatoes are a fruit that's very often overlooked. Most people don't even think it's a fruit...but it is.

I would even call it a super-fruit. It's rich in alkaline minerals and very low in sugar. It's hydrating and tastes great in salads, soups, smoothies, and juices.

Tomato juice offers potent antioxidant properties and phytonutrients that defend your body from free radicals that cause damage to your cells.

It also makes your skin look younger, healthier, and more glowing. There are many more benefits...Tomato juice makes an excellent workout recovery drink, helping your body stay in balance.

Recipe #6 "It Doesn't Have to Be Gross" Nourishment Juice

Beets are rich in antioxidants and anti-inflammatory phytonutrients, like betalains. Moreover, beetroot is also a diuretic, helping fight water retention, edema, and cellulite. So, if you don't like eating beets, juice them. Personally, I prefer the second option.

When juiced with other ingredients, such as carrots and limes, beets create a potent natural drink. Thanks to beets and cinnamon, it has an original and a slightly sweet flavor.

Servings: 2
Ingredients:
- 4 beets, peeled
- 4 carrots, peeled and cut into smaller pieces
- 2 limes, peeled
- 1 apple, cut into smaller pieces
- A pinch of cinnamon and nutmeg powder
- half cup coconut milk (or other nut or plant-based milk of your choice)
- 1 tablespoon avocado or flaxseed oil (optional)

Instructions:

1. Juice the beets, carrots, limes, and apple using a juicer.
1. Now, stir in the cinnamon and nutmeg powder.
2. Finally, stir in the coconut milk and avocado or flaxseed oil.
3. Serve and enjoy. To your health!

Recipe #7 "Minty Digestion Tonic" Juice

This recipe helps maintain a healthy digestive system and strengthens your immune system with vitamin C and the healing properties of ginger. It's a fantastic way to make a tasty, energizing water to help you stay healthy and hydrated. Plain water can get boring, so try this tonic juice recipe...

Servings: 2

Ingredients:

- 1 fennel bulb (it's optional, so don't worry if you can't find one)
- 4 grapefruits, peeled and chopped
- 2 inches of ginger, peeled
- 4 cups of water
- A few orange slices
- Optional: stevia to sweeten if needed

Instructions:

1. Place all the ingredients through a juicer to extract the juice, reserving the orange slices.
2. Pour the juice in a jar and mix it with water.
3. Add in a few orange slices.
4. Serve chilled with some ice cubes.
5. Enjoy!

Fennel bulb is one of the best ingredients for non-green alkaline juicing. It's naturally sweet and will give your juices and tonics a fantastic flavor. It's an excellent natural remedy to help you take care of your immune system. It contains a lot of vitamin C, potassium (an alkaline electrolyte), and it's rich in an inflammation-reducing phytonutrient called anethole.

Recipe #8 "Coconut Hydration" Empowerment Juice

You can't juice coconut. Just like you can't juice bananas or avocados. But...you can still enjoy a sweet coconut flavor in your non-green juices by mixing them with some coconut milk.

If you are allergic to coconut milk or can't find it, feel free to use any other healthy plant-based milk of your choice (just make sure you stay away from brands that add sugar or other nasty stuff to their products).

The main ingredients here are fennel bulb and zucchini. Just like cucumber, zucchini technically is green, but it doesn't taste green, and it's certainly not so green when peeled.

One of the main benefits of juicing zucchini is taking advantage is its high nutrient profile (vitamin A and C, manganese, vitamin C, potassium, and magnesium) and high level of antioxidants to help you have beautiful skin and healthy eyes.

Servings: 2
Ingredients:
- 4 big zucchinis, slightly peeled
- 1 lime, peeled and chopped
- 2 yellow or red bell peppers
- 1 tablespoon coconut oil, melted
- Himalayan salt to taste, if needed
- Half cup thick coconut milk

Instructions:

1. Put the zucchinis, lime, and peppers through a juicer.
2. Extract the juice.
3. Pour into a chilled glass.
4. Add in the coconut oil and coconut milk.
5. Season with Himalayan salt if needed.
6. Enjoy!

Recipe #9 "Create Your Balance" Energy Juice

Radish is a powerful source of vitamin C and potassium. It tastes great in juices, especially when balanced out by a naturally sweet red bell pepper.

Maca is a natural hormone balancer for women, and you can add it to this juice too (it's optional though).

Coconut milk and coconut oil not only add more nutrients and amazing flavor, but they also add to the volume of this fantastic drink so that you can enjoy sipping on it longer!

Servings: 2
Ingredients:
- Half cup radish
- 1 inch of ginger, peeled
- 2 red bell peppers
- 1 tablespoon coconut oil (optional)
- 1 cup coconut milk (or any other healthy nut or plant-based milk of your choice)
- Half teaspoon maca powder
- Cinnamon and nutmeg powder to taste

Instructions:
1. Juice the radish, ginger, and peppers using a juicer.
2. Pour into a glass.
3. Add the rest of the ingredients.
4. Stir well, serve and enjoy!

Recipe #10 "I Don't Have the Time to Juice" Easy Juice

This recipe is perfect if you are too busy to juice using a juicer. Or perhaps the mere thought of setting up your Omega juicer and doing proper juicing makes you procrastinate.

The good news is that you can still keep going with your healthy juicing routine. And you don't need anything fancy. Just stay committed to the process!

This recipe doesn't even need a proper juicer. A simple lemon squeezer will do. This simple recipe helps detoxify the liver; it works really well first thing in the morning.

Serves: 1
Ingredients:
- 2 lemons, juiced
- 1 cup of coconut water
- 1 teaspoon avocado oil

Instructions:
1. Juice the lemons using a lemon squeezer.
2. In a glass, combine the lemon juice with the coconut water and avocado oil.
3. Stir well and drink.
4. To your health! Enjoy!

Recipe #11 "Replenish Yourself" Juice

Coconut water can be a fantastic addition to your juicing recipes. It's excellent for optimal hydration, full of alkaline minerals to help your body stay in balance. It also offers natural sweetness, which is something that may be needed for recipes rich in citric fruit such as grapefruit.

Whenever I feel like I am coming down with the flu, or simply need to give my body more rest and nourishment, I turn to this recipe. It's pretty quick to make, too and it doesn't require hours spent on juicing.

Serves: 2-3
Ingredients:
- 1 cup coconut water
- 2-inch ginger
- 1 garlic clove, peeled
- 5 grapefruits
- Optional- stevia to sweeten

Instructions:
1. Juice the ginger, garlic, and grapefruit.
2. Combine with coconut water and ice cubes.
3. Sweeten with a little stevia if you like.
4. Serve and enjoy!

Recipe #12 "Red Pepper Detox" Juice

Fennel and mint help create a sweet flavor while contributing more healing nutrients to help you thrive.

Red bell peppers are one of my favorite non-green juicing ingredients. Not only do they taste great, but they are also jam-packed with nutrients, such as vitamin C, vitamin A, as well as vitamin E, vitamin K, vitamin B6, niacin, potassium, magnesium, and riboflavin.

With such a mighty army of nutrients, red bell pepper juice is excellent as a natural antioxidant, holistic beauty remedy (great for general wellbeing, beautiful skin, and improved energy) as well as a healthy cardiovascular system.

When juicing red bell peppers, you can keep the pulp and add it to your curries, stir-fries, and other veggie dishes.

Servings: 2
Ingredients:
- 4 big red bell peppers
- 1 fennel bulb
- A handful of mint leaves (optional)
- Half cup of coconut milk
- 1 tablespoon avocado oil
- Optional- stevia to sweeten

Instructions:
1. Juice the peppers, fennel, and mint.
2. Add the coconut milk and avocado oil.
3. Stir well, adding stevia if needed.
4. Enjoy!

Recipe #13 "Liver Lover" Juice

The combination of ingredients from this recipe helps heal the liver while helping you enjoy more energy, balance, and zest for life.

As weird as it may sound, especially for beginners, grapefruits and lemons are one of the most alkaline fruits ever (even though the taste is acidic, which can be a bit confusing for beginners). It's because they are very low in sugar and high in alkaline nutrients.

When it comes to healthy juicing, it's essential to focus on low sugar fruits. Even if you are not interested in the alkaline diet, it still makes sense, right?

Sugar (even natural) can be one of those secret enemies stealing away your energy and vitality. Another reason to add more lemons and grapefruits to your diet is the fantastic benefits that they offer.

Grapefruit Benefits:
- Rich in phytonutrients called limonoids that promote the production of antioxidant enzymes. These help the liver to remove toxic compounds easier, thereby protecting the liver in the process.

Lemon Benefits:
- Also rich in limonoids, lemons take care of liver function by strengthening liver enzymes, as well as regulating blood carbohydrate levels.

Servings: 2-4
Ingredients:
- 2 grapefruits, peeled
- 2 lemons, peeled
- 1 garlic clove, peeled (optional)
- 1 inch of fresh root ginger, peeled
- Half cup water, filtered, preferably alkaline
- 1 tablespoon of Udo's Choice (you can also use cold-pressed flax oil)
- Pinch of Himalayan salt

Instructions:
1. Juice the grapefruits, lemons, garlic, and ginger.
2. Add the water, Udo's Choice, and Himalayan salt.
3. Stir well and drink to your health.

Grapefruit Benefits:
- Rich in phytonutrients called limonoids that promote the production of antioxidant enzymes. These help the liver remove the toxic compounds more easily, thereby protecting the liver in the process.

Lemon Benefits:
- Also rich in limonoids, lemons take care of the liver function by strengthening liver enzymes, as well as regulating blood carbohydrate levels.

Recipe #14 "Super Buzz" Body and Mind Energizing Juice

Who wants more energy? Right here, right now? Well, energy is just in front of you!

What I really like about this recipe is its natural creaminess thanks to cashew milk.

Personally, I like combining my juices (especially non-green juices where the ingredient list is a bit limited) with delicious and nutritious kinds of nut milk for more taste and variety.

Servings: 2-3
Ingredients:
- 2 cucumbers, peeled
- 1-inch ginger, peeled
- 1-inch turmeric, peeled
- Half fennel bulb
- 2 yellow bell peppers
- 1 tablespoon olive or avocado oil
- 1 cup of raw cashew milk (unsweetened) or coconut milk
- Pinch of black pepper

Instructions:
1. Wash all the veggies.
2. Chop and juice them, adding ginger and turmeric.
3. Stir in some olive or avocado oil and mix in the cashew milk and pepper.
4. Drink immediately.
5. Enjoy the energy!

Recipe #15 "Wake Up Maca Juice"

Fresh alkaline juices are natural energy boosters; however, by adding some maca powder, we can really take it to the next level!

Maca is a plant native to Peru that in recent years has gained a lot of popularity in health and wellness communities. It is usually taken as a powdered supplement or in capsules.

It's jam-packed with nutrients such as vitamin C, copper, potassium, iron, manganese and vitamin B6. It's commonly used as an aphrodisiac for both men and women, as well as a natural remedy and mood booster for menopausal women.

Athletes and high performers also love using maca as a natural supplement to boost energy and increase physical and mental performance. Personally, I love putting maca powder in my smoothies (or tea) before extended writing or content creation sessions.

As with many natural supplements and remedies that I recommend, maca is generally considered safe. However, if you are on medication, have experienced any serious health issues, are pregnant or lactating, have thyroid problems (or simply want to be confident knowing that this natural remedy is safe for you) I highly recommend that you talk to your doctor first.

Servings: 2-3
Ingredients:
- 6 big tomatoes
- A few fennel slices
- 1-inch ginger, peeled
- Half cup radish
- 1 lemon, peeled
- Half teaspoon of maca powder
- 1 teaspoon olive oil or avocado oil (ootional)
- A pinch of Himalayan salt

Instructions:
1. Wash and chop the tomatoes, fennel, ginger, radish, and lemon.
2. Put through a juicer to extract their juices.
3. Pour the juice into a tall glass and add some maca powder.
4. Add some olive or avocado oil and a bit of Himalayan salt.
5. Stir well, serve and enjoy!

Recipe #16 "Boost Your Metabolism" Juice

Small actions and consistency lead to significant transformations. You don't need anything fancy or too complicated. Simply focus on nutrient-dense foods and try to have at least one alkaline juice a day. This recipe offers a unique taste, pH balancing properties, metabolism-boosting properties, and is also great for your skin.

Servings: 1-2
Ingredients:
- 2 large grapefruits, peeled
- 2 big carrots, peeled, unless organic
- 1 orange, peeled
- 1-inch ginger, peeled
- Half cup coconut or almond milk

Instructions:
1. Push the grapefruits, carrots, orange, and ginger through a juicer.
2. Add some coconut or almond milk and stir well.
3. Drink immediately.
4. Enjoy!

Recipe #17 "Colorful Energy" Detox Juice

Beets are a fantastic source of potassium, a mineral electrolyte that helps nerves and muscles function correctly. It's also rich in vitamin C as well as a myriad of minerals such as calcium, iron, magnesium, manganese, phosphorus, sodium, zinc, copper, and selenium. Everything you need to enjoy more energy and vitality! In one juicing session, you can enjoy more nutrients than a fast-food eating person gets in a week or even a month...

And those small healthy decisions always add up...

This recipe is jam-packed with minerals and vital nutrients. Lemon and lime add more flavor to this juice and make it a great, refreshing drink for any time of the day.

Servings: 1-2
Ingredients:
- 2 medium cucumbers, peeled
- 2 beetroots, peeled
- 2 lemons, peeled
- 1 lime, peeled
- 1 teaspoon olive oil or avocado oil (optional)
- Pinch of Himalayan salt

Instructions:
1. Put the cucumbers, beets, lemons, and lime through a juicer.
2. When ready, pour the juice in a juice glass or another utensil of your choice and stir in a pinch of Himalayan salt and olive oil (or any other quality cold-pressed oil of your choice). Good fats help your body with nutrient absorption. Enjoy!

Recipe #18 "Spicy Red Bell Pepper" Juice

Feeling a bit peckish between meals? Nothing to worry about. Listen to your body and give it some vital nutrients! This is what it needs. And this is why it is sending you the "Feed me; I need some awesome nutrients for energy so that I can work for you!" signals.

This juice uses a bit of basil (yes, I know, a green ingredient that just sneaked in) to add to the taste and aroma of this juice.

You can always skip it, though!

Servings: 1-2
Ingredients:
- 4 big red bell peppers
- 4 cucumbers (peeled)
- 2 big tomatoes
- 1 lime, peeled
- A handful of fresh basil leaves (optional)
- A couple of drops of Tabasco (optional)
- Pinch of Himalayan salt
- 1 tablespoon of olive oil or any other quality cold-pressed oil

Instructions:

1. Put the peppers, cucumber, tomatoes, lime, and basil through a juicer.
2. When the juice is ready, stir in some Tabasco (according to your taste preferences, but trust me, this

juice is excellent as a spicy one), oil of your choice, and Himalayan salt.

3. Enjoy!

Additional Information:

Sweet Peppers (orange, yellow, and red) protect your skin against sunburn and are good for the heart. They also have a pleasant, sweet-like taste and always make an excellent snack between meals. They are nutrient-packed as they are rich in beta carotene, vitamin C, folate, B1, B2, B3, B5, B6, vitamin E, vitamin K, iron, and manganese. If you like sweeter juices and want to avoid juicing sugary fruit (not the best thing to do anyway), start juicing sweet peppers (all except green peppers are sweet).

Basil is an excellent herb that will give your juices a lovely flavor. It is superbly antiseptic, antibacterial, as well as fungicidal. It's great for digestion. It is rich in beta carotene, vitamin C, folate, B1, B2, B3, B5, B6, vitamin E, copper, magnesium, potassium, iron, manganese, phosphorus, calcium, zinc, and even some omega 3. I always say there is no need to splurge on super-expensive and exotic superfoods. The best alkaline superfoods are usually very easy to get.

Recipe #19 "Spicy Ginger Vitamin C Juice" for Natural Energy

This simple juice recipe offers a fantastic combination of ginger and lemon juice with spices and nut milk.

You can enjoy this simple recipe super-chilled or slightly warm (perfect as a warming pick me up drink in the winter).

Servings: 2
Ingredients:
- 4 lemons, peeled
- 4-inch ginger, peeled
- 1-inch turmeric
- 1 cup coconut or cashew milk
- Half teaspoon cinnamon powder
- Half teaspoon vanilla powder
- Half teaspoon nutmeg powder
- Pinch of black pepper
- Stevia to sweeten (optional)
- 1 teaspoon coconut oil

Instructions:
1. Juice the lemons, ginger, and turmeric.
2. Combine with coconut or cashew milk, coconut oil, and spices.
3. If needed, sweeten with stevia.
4. Stir well, serve and enjoy!

***If serving this drink in the winter, heat your milk so that it's warm (but not boiling) before you combine it with the juice.

Recipe #20 "Light Alkaline Keto Smoothie-Style" Juice

This recipe is a bit different as it combines juicing with blending. It's very rich in vitamins A and C to help you have beautiful skin and a healthy immune system while enjoying more energy.

This smoothie-style juice is particularly useful for healthy eyesight and beautiful skin as it is packed with vitamins A and C. It also uses avocado and chia seeds to fill you up and revitalize your body with good fats and clean calories.

Ingredients:
For the Juice:
- 2 red bell peppers
- Half cup radish
- 2 big tomatoes
- 1-inch ginger
- 1 lime, peeled

For the Smoothie:

- Half an avocado, peeled and pitted
- Half cup coconut or cashew milk (raw and unsweetened)
- 1 tablespoon chia seeds
- Half teaspoon maca

Instructions:
1. First juice all the juicing ingredients by placing red bell peppers, radish, tomatoes, ginger, and lime through a juicer.
2. Place the juice in a blender and add the avocado, cashew or coconut milk, chia seeds, and maca powder.
3. Blend well until smooth.
4. Stir well, serve and enjoy!

Avocados cannot be juiced (unfortunately), so the only way to incorporate them into your juices is to blend them in.

While the process of combining juicing with blending is a bit more time consuming, it's totally worth it!

Avocados are incredibly nutritious (vitamin K, folate, vitamin C, potassium, vitamin B5, and B6, as well as vitamin E) and loaded with healthy fats and fiber. They are also very rich in potassium (to support healthy blood pressure levels).

Adding avocados or avocado oil to your juices (as well as salads and smoothies) helps the nutrients you take in absorb faster.

And yes, avocados are green, but they don't taste green. We are using them to add some good fats to our diets.

Recipe #21 "Release Toxins and Fat" Juice

This recipe fuses low sugar alkaline fruits with horsetail infusion. Horsetail infusion is an excellent natural remedy to help you get rid of water retention, lose weight, and burn fat. It's full of alkaline minerals and blends really well with this juice.

Once again, since the non-green alkaline green juice ingredient list is a bit limited, it's good to get creative.

Combining your juices with herbal infusions, or, as I previously suggested, delicious creamy nut milk (or both) makes the whole process more exciting and fun.

Serves: 2-3
Ingredients:
- 1 tablespoon of fresh mint leaves
- 1 grapefruit, peeled
- 1 lime, peeled
- Half inch ginger, peeled
- 2 big carrots, peeled
- Half cup horsetail infusion, cooled
- Half cup coconut milk
- Half teaspoon cinnamon powder
- Half teaspoon coconut oil
- Optional: stevia to sweeten

Instructions:
1. First, juice the mint, grapefruit, lime, ginger, and carrots.
2. Combine with horsetail infusion and coconut milk.
3. Add the cinnamon powder and stevia if needed.

4. Add the coconut oil.
5. Serve and enjoy!

Recipe #22 "Detox While You Sleep" Non-Green Alkaline Juice

This delicious herbal juice uses verbena- a herb used to stimulate relaxation and peace of mind.

Servings: 1-2
Ingredients:
- 1 cup of verbena infusion, cooled down a bit (use 1 teabag per cup)
- 2 grapefruits, peeled and sliced
- 1 cup of coconut milk
- 1 tablespoon of fresh mint leaves
- Stevia to sweeten, if needed

Instructions:
1. Juice the grapefruits and mint leaves.
2. Mix the juice with the infusion and the coconut milk.
3. Stir well and add stevia for naturally sweet taste.
4. Enjoy!

Verbena is a pretty safe herb, but there is not enough information to confirm whether it can be used during pregnancy or breastfeeding. The same applies to possible contraindications with other medications. I always recommend consulting with your doctor first.

Recipe #23 "Beat the Sugar Cravings" Juice

This recipe will help you get rid of sugar cravings while feeding your body with a myriad of nutrients it needs to thrive. Pomegranate juice is full of alkaline minerals, as well as vitamin C.

It's a natural antioxidant and anti-inflammatory. It blends really well with ginger and turmeric, creating a fantastic color and taste.

Servings: 2
Ingredients:
- 1 cup pomegranate seeds
- 1-inch ginger root, peeled
- 1-inch turmeric root, peeled
- 1 tablespoon of avocado oil
- Pinch of black pepper
- Stevia to sweeten (optional)

Instructions:
1. Juice the pomegranate seeds, ginger, and turmeric.
2. Combine with avocado oil and black pepper.
3. If needed, sweeten with stevia.
4. Serve and enjoy!

Recipe #24 Simple "Mojito Style" Juice

It's time for a simple and super-nutritious, non-alcoholic version of mojito!

Servings: 2-3
Ingredients:
- 4 cucumbers, peeled and sliced
- 3 cups alkaline (or filtered) water
- Stevia to sweeten (optional)

To Garnish:
- A few mint leaves to garnish
- A few lime slices to garnish
- Half cup ice cubes
- Stevia to sweeten

Instructions:
1. Juice the cucumbers.
2. Pour the fresh juice into a tall water jar or pitcher.
3. Add water and ice cubes.
4. Now, add the mint leaves and lime slices.
5. If needed, sweeten with stevia.
6. Stir in well, chill in the fridge for a few hours, and serve.
7. Enjoy!

Recipe #25 "Unlimited Energy" Juice

While it's hard to eat a mountain of veggies, it's easy to drink their juice and get all the vital nutrients from them. The energy you get is almost instant. And the more you do it, the better you feel! Avocado oil offers good fat to help you absorb the minerals and vitamins from the juice.

Servings: 2
Ingredients:
- 4 big red bell peppers
- 2 limes, peeled
- 1 lemon, peeled
- 2 tablespoons of avocado oil
- Himalayan salt and black pepper to taste

Instructions:
1. Put the peppers, limes, and lemon through a juicer.
2. Pour into a glass and mix in some Himalayan salt and black pepper to taste. Stir in the avocado oil.
3. Enjoy!

Recipe #26 Spicy Coconut Drink

While pure beetroot juice can be a bit hardcore, this recipe is a little different as it uses coconut milk and delicious spices. It's very nutritious and rich in good fats. And yes, you still get all the benefits of drinking vegetable juice while enjoying natural sweetness and creaminess.

Serves: 2

Ingredients:

- 2 cups of fresh beet slices
- 2-inch ginger, peeled
- 1 cup coconut milk, unsweetened
- 1 tablespoon coconut oil (optional)
- 1 teaspoon cinnamon powder
- Pinch of nutmeg powder
- Optional: stevia to sweeten

Instructions:

1. Put the beets and ginger through a juicer.
2. Extract the juice, pour it in a big glass.
3. Add some melted coconut oil, coconut milk, spices, and stevia.
4. Stir well and enjoy!

Recipe #27 "Red and Spicy" Juice

Tomato, ginger, and healthful oils make an excellent combination.

Italian herbs take it to the next level! Once again, alkaline juices can be tasty, exciting, and fun.

Servings: 2
Ingredients:
- 8 big organic tomatoes, chopped
- 2 inches of ginger, peeled
- 2 garlic cloves, peeled
- 1 teaspoon organic olive oil (optional)
- 1 teaspoon dried Italian/ Mediterranean herbs (whatever you choose: oregano, thyme, rosemary)
- Himalayan salt to taste

Instructions:
1. Juice the tomatoes, ginger and garlic using a juicer.
2. Combine with olive oil.
3. Add Himalayan salt and herbs.
4. Enjoy!

Recipe #28 Simple Alkaline Energy Drink

While I definitely don't promote the idea of juicing sugary fruits, it's absolutely fine to add a bit of apple to your juice now and again to make it taste sweeter.

It's all about balance and common sense.

Anything too restrictive borders on a dietary cult, which is something I am not a fan of!

Servings: 2
Ingredients:
- 2 green apples, peeled and chopped
- 1 lemon, peeled and halved
- 4 carrots, peeled
- 1 inch of ginger, peeled
- 1-inch turmeric, peeled
- 1 teaspoon avocado oil
- Pinch of black pepper

Instructions:
1. Juice the apples, lemon, carrots, ginger, and turmeric in a juicer.
2. Stir in the avocado oil and pepper.
3. Serve in a glass.
4. Enjoy!

Recipe #29 Easy Light Juice

This is a super-hydrating, alkalizing juice with a fresh, light, citrus flavor.

Servings: 2
Ingredients:
- 4 medium cucumbers, peeled and chopped
- 4 grapefruits, peeled
- 1 cup water, filtered, preferably alkaline
- 1 cup coconut water for natural sweetness
- Ice cubes (optional)

Instructions:
1. Put the cucumbers and grapefruits through a juicer.
2. Extract the juice.
3. Mix with water and coconut water.
4. Pour into a chilled water jar and stir well.
5. Serve in a glass with some ice cubes.

This recipe is one of my favorite morning drinks during hot summers. It's excellent for getting almost instant energy and is super-hydrating. You already know that drinking water in the morning is good for you and is an excellent morning ritual for health, energy, and focus.

Well, this recipe will help you take it to the next level. Not only are you hydrating your body, mind, and soul, but you're also nourishing yourself with alkaline minerals and vitamins. Try it! It's also a fantastic replenishment drink after working out. It also helps you concentrate better and be more productive.

Recipe #30 Naturally Sweet Energy Juice

Red bell peppers are one of my favorite veggies to juice. They are naturally sweet and full of vitamins and minerals. They make any juice taste amazing!

In this recipe, they blend with green and fennel tea to help you stay energized.

Quite an unusual combo, isn't it?

Servings: 2
Ingredients:
- 3 red bell peppers, seeded and chopped
- 1 inch of ginger, peeled
- 1 lime, peeled
- 1 cup of green tea and fennel tea (combine 1 cup of boiling water with 1 green tea bag and 1 fennel tea bag)

Instructions:
1. Juice the peppers, ginger and lime using a juicer.
2. Set aside.
3. Make the tea and cool it down.
4. Now, combine the tea with the juice.
5. Stir well, serve and enjoy!

This recipe can be a great mid-morning or afternoon pick me up. If you are having this drink in the afternoon, you may want to get rid of green tea, especially if you tend to suffer from insomnia, or if caffeine-containing drinks make you nervous. This drink also works amazingly without green tea.

Recipe #31 Easy Coconut Energy Boosting Mix

Compared to other juicing recipes, this one is relatively simple and quick to make as it leverages the coconut water. Just perfect as a quick, energy-boosting juice.

Servings: 2
Ingredients:
- 4 big carrots, peeled and chopped
- 2 green apples, chopped
- 2-inch ginger, peeled
- 1 cup of coconut water, unsweetened
- 1 teaspoon avocado oil (optional)

Instructions:
1. Juice the carrots, apples, and ginger.
2. Pour into a glass and mix with 1 cup of coconut water.
3. Stir well, add in the avocado oil.
4. Stir well again, serve and enjoy!

Recipe #32 Simple Vitamin C Juice

This recipe is very quick and easy to make, even without a juicer.

Servings: 2
Ingredients:
- 2 big grapefruits, halved horizontally to squeeze the juice
- 2 lemons, halved horizontally to squeeze the juice
- Pinch of Himalayan salt
- 1 teaspoon avocado oil

Instructions:
1. Juice the grapefruits and lemons (a lemon squeezer tool, like the one in the picture below, will do for this recipe).
2. Combine the juice with avocado oil and salt.
3. Stir well, serve in a glass and enjoy!

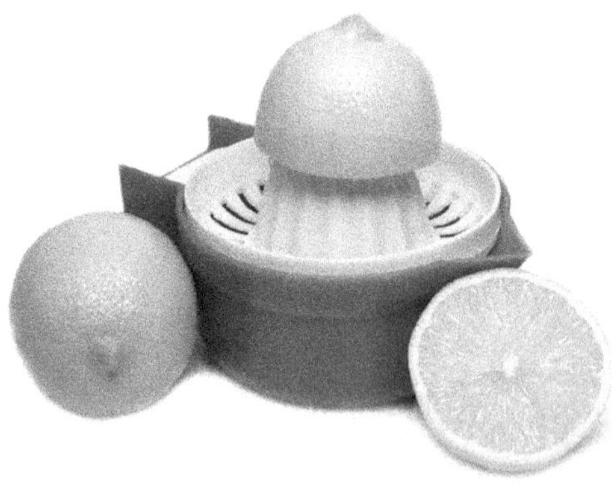

Recipe #33 Bullet Proof Green Tea and Vitamin C Juice

This recipe uses green tea to help you boost your energy levels and burn fat. Ginger adds to its anti-inflammatory properties. Then, there is grapefruit which is rich in vitamin C and alkaline minerals. That mix combines really well with coconut oil. So tasty and good for you!

Servings: 2
Ingredients:
- 1 big grapefruit
- 2-inch ginger, peeled
- 2-inch turmeric, peeled
- 1 cup green tea, cooled (use 1 teabag per cup)
- 1 tablespoon coconut oil (optional)
- Pinch of black pepper
- Stevia to sweeten if needed

Instructions:
1. Make the green tea and leave covered to cool down.
2. In the meantime, juice the grapefruits, ginger, and turmeric.
3. Combine the tea with the juice, adding the coconut oil and black pepper (to help with turmeric absorption).
4. Stir well, and if needed, add stevia.

Grapefruit juice benefits:
-helps in weight loss (it's low in calories and high in nutrients)
-very low in carbs and sugars
-stimulates the lymphatic system, helping you feel lighter and more energized
-boosts the immune system

Recipe #34 "Beta Carotene Powerhouse" for Healthy-Looking Skin

This juice is a fantastic combination of tomatoes, turmeric, and ginger to help you have beautiful and healthy-looking skin while enjoying more natural energy.

It's also great as a quick apéritif and it provides nourishment for more energy.

Servings: 2
Ingredients:
- 6 big tomatoes, chopped
- 2-inch turmeric, peeled
- 2-inch ginger, peeled
- 2 tablespoons olive oil
- Pinch of Himalayan salt
- Pinch of black pepper

Instructions:
1. Juice the tomatoes, turmeric and ginger.
2. Pour into a glass and add in the olive oil, Himalayan salt and black pepper.
3. Enjoy!

Recipe #35 A Restorative Antioxidant Non-Green Juice

This juice shows once again that healthy juicing can go beyond juicing greens. Yellow bell peppers blend very well with grapefruits and ginger.

Servings: 2
Ingredients:
- 4 big yellow bell peppers, cut into smaller pieces
- 1-inch ginger, peeled
- 2 big grapefruits, peeled and cut into smaller pieces
- 1 teaspoon avocado oil

Instructions:
1. Juice the peppers, ginger and grapefruits.
2. Combine with avocado oil.
3. Serve in a big glass and enjoy!

Yellow bell peppers are an excellent natural antioxidant, and a very rich source of potassium (to enhance muscle strength and regulate fluid balance) as well as vitamin C for a strong, healthy immune system.

They are also very rich in luteolin, a compound known to reduce the signs of stress and anger. Another compound they offer, quercetin, helps you unwind and reduce stress.

Conclusion – Healthy Lifestyle Tips

Here are a few simple guidelines that will help you transition towards a healthy, alkaline lifestyle. These are compatible with different nutritional lifestyles (Gluten Free, Vegetarian, Vegan, Keto, Paleo) and it's totally up to you what you choose to focus on:

Eliminate processed foods from your diet and say "no" to colas and sodas

There are so many additives and preservatives in these foods. They have been known to create hormone imbalances, make you tired, and add to acidity in your body. It's just not natural for humans to consume those conveniently processed foods.

The label may even say "low in calories or low in fat" but it will not help you in your long-term weight loss or health efforts. In order to start losing weight naturally, your body needs foods that are jam-packed with nutrients. Real foods. Living foods.

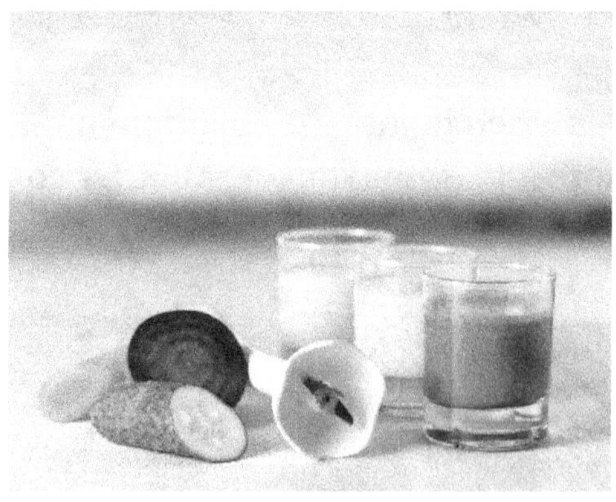

Drink plenty of clean, filtered water

Preferably drink alkaline water or alkaline fruit-infused water (lemons, grapefruits, limes and pomegranates are great for that).

Add more vegetable juices into your diet

These are a great way to give your body more nutrients and alkalinity that will result in more energy, less inflammation and, if desired, natural weight loss.

Vegetable juices are the best shots of health! I have also written a book called *Alkaline Juicing* if you want to give it a try and want to learn how to juice the right way, to enjoy more energy and health.

Reduce/eliminate processed grains, "crappy carbs" as well as yeast (very acid forming).

Personally, I recommend quinoa instead (it's naturally gluten-free), some sweet potatoes or some fresh seasonal fruit.

You can also use gluten-free wraps or make your own bread.

Reduce caffeine

As long as you have a healthy foundation, you can have coffee as a treat (I do drink coffee occasionally, or when I have to wake up very early; or when I meet up with a friend, "for a coffee").

There is no reason to be too strict on yourself, just don't rely on caffeine as your main source of energy. Green tea may be helpful too as a transition, but green tea is not caffeine-free either so don't overdo it.

On the other end of the spectrum - green tea is rich in antioxidants and a great part of a balanced diet, so it's not that you have to get paranoid about all kinds of caffeine. Moderation is the key.

Try to observe your body. Personally, I have noticed that quitting my coffee habits (I used to have 2-3 coffees a day) and replacing coffee with natural herbal teas and infusions has really made my energy levels skyrocket.

Now I sleep better, and I get up feeling nice and fresh. I don't need caffeine to keep me awake. I no longer suffer from tension headaches and I feel calmer.

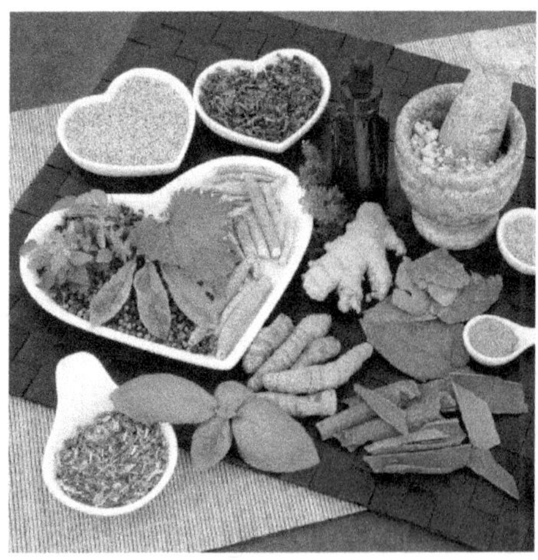

You can use stevia instead of processed sugar and Himalayan salt instead of regular salt - Stevia is sweet but sugar-free and Himalayan salt contains calcium, iron, potassium and magnesium plus it also contains lower amounts of sodium than regular salt.

Add more spices and herbs to your diet- not only do they make your dishes taste amazing, but they also have anti-inflammatory properties and help you detoxify (cilantro, turmeric, and cinnamon are miraculous).

As you can see, the Alkaline Diet is a pretty common-sense clean diet. Nothing is exaggerated. Nothing is too strict. Nothing is too faddish. Eat more living foods and avoid processed foods. Try to eat more plant-based foods (even if you're not fully vegan).

Add regular relaxation techniques to the Alkaline Diet (including yoga, meditation), time spent in nature, adequate sleep and physical activity (we need to sweat out those toxins) and you have a prescription for holistic wellbeing!

This is the gist of the Alkaline Diet lifestyle. This is what will make you feel fresh and rejuvenated and help you achieve your ideal weight. The problem is that some people are not willing to take those small common-sense steps and are looking for a "secret formula"- something that will magically help them with no effort at all. I am not judging- I have been guilty of it as well. We all have!

The truth is that whatever changes you want to make in your life (this rule applies not only to health) can be hard. Leaving one's comfort zone is difficult, but with time and practice it becomes easy and automatic.

Holistic success is about applying what we already know and using the information to better our lives. This is what I call "the secret formula." <u>Information in action</u>. I always say that I am very open-minded when it comes to different diets. I never claim that what I do is the only path to wellness and health. I prefer to provide you with information and inspiration so that you can create your own way and choose what works for you. Everyone is different.

You need to learn to listen to your body and be good to yourself.

Everyone is different, which is why your alkaline lifestyle will be different to mine. However, many elements remain similar, and it is my hope that this book has given you the tools, recipes and inspiration you need to be successful on your health and wellness quest.

Feel free to come back to this book whenever you need more motivation.

It's all about making consistent progress and about those small daily decisions.

They will help you create what I like to call *empowering alkaline mini habits*. These, when compounded, will help you to transform in a way you never even thought was possible. It will be an amazing experience.

Finally, I need to ask you for a small favor. It will only take a few minutes of your precious time and will be very helpful for me at this stage. All I am asking you for is your honest review on Amazon. Your review, even a short one, can inspire someone else to start living a healthy lifestyle and enjoy the benefits of juicing!

Let's make this world a happy, healthy and more empowered place.

That collective transformation starts with small baby steps and micro-actions.

Thank you, thank you, thank you.

Marta

About Marta

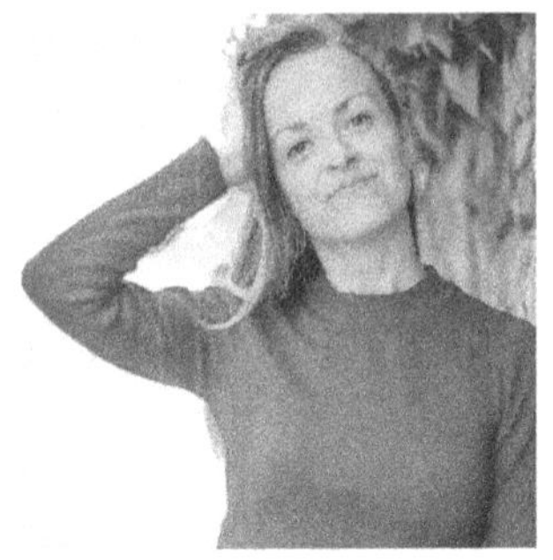

Marta Tuchowska is a serial author, creative entrepreneur and wellness advocate with a background in several natural/ holistic wellness modalities (certified in holistic nutrition, aromatherapy, and Reiki) and motivational/lifestyle coaching.

She's very passionate about creating simple-to-follow wellness and recipe books aimed at empowering her readers to take care of their wellbeing in a truly holistic way. All systems must go- mind, body and soul! It's all about taking those small, daily actions that lead to big transformations.

You can connect with Marta by emailing her at:

martaholisticwellness@gmail.com

or info@holisticwellnessproject.com

To join Marta's mailing list, visit:

www.HolisticWellnessProject.com/alkaline

Similar Books Written by Marta

(now available on Amazon)

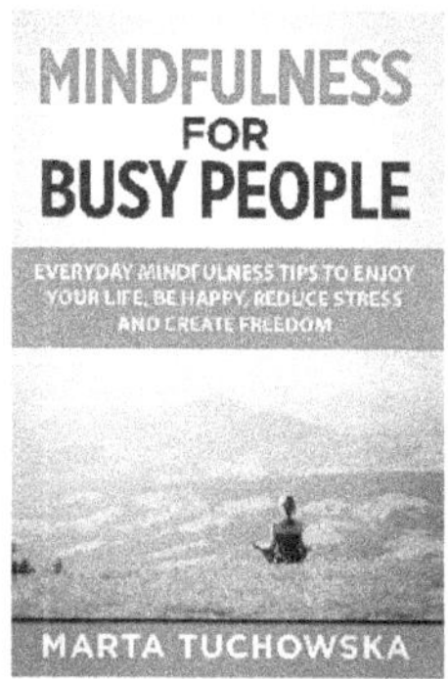

Mindfulness for Busy People: Everyday Mindfulness Tips to Enjoy Your Life, Be Happy, Reduce Stress and Create Freedom

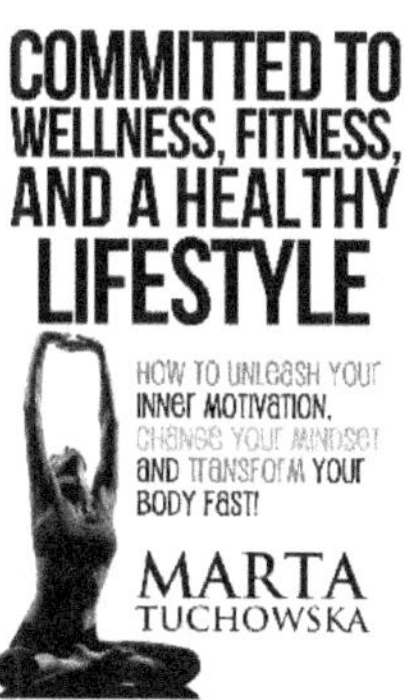

Committed to Wellness, Fitness, and a Healthy Lifestyle: How to Unleash Your Inner Motivation, Change Your Mindset, and Transform Your Body Fast